Dave's Thin Book on Weight Loss

DAVID D. MICKELSON

Disclaimer:

The information provided in this book should not be construed as personal medical advice or instruction. Readers should consult appropriate health professionals on any matter relating to their health and well being.

Dedication

This book is dedicated to my wife, my children and my grandchildren. After achieving a healthy weight, I am able to enjoy a more active lifestyle and for many more years than otherwise would have been the case. Time spent with my family is a precious gift.

About the Author

I am not a personal trainer, I am not a nutritionist, and I am not a celebrity. My only credentials are the success of my own personal weight loss program–a physically fit body, and the loss of over forty five pounds in the span of eighteen months.

The principles contained in this book have changed my life in many positive ways. My sincere hope is that it does the same for you. Have a great and happy life!

Index

Dave's Thin Book on Weight Loss

E very essential change in a person's life begins with a **pivotal moment**. Mine happened when I looked in the mirror one morning and my breast size was starting to rival that of my wife's. Now couple that with an incessant snoring problem, due to excess weight, that was forcing my wife to sleep in a separate bedroom and—well, you get the picture.

The pathway to a healthier life requires a healthy weight. There are thousands of weight-loss books and tapes in the world that will thoroughly instruct you on how to lose that weight. If you don't believe me, go to a garage sale sometime. There are books on weight loss, tapes on weight loss, CDs on weight loss, video tapes on weight loss, DVDs on weight loss—maybe even a reel-to-reels on weight loss—and all of them stacked next to the exercise bike or stair climber they were going to use next week. The fact is you have to want to be at a better weight, and you have to do something about it. What you do must make sense, and have a goal of sustainable weight loss in order to reach that ideal body weight for you. Why are most dieting books fat like your waistline? It is because they present a complicated formula for success while covering every imaginable detail. How many truly complicated things have you accomplished in your life? Simplify the process and you increase the potential for success. The following information is just that! It is not a formula. It is not calorie counting. It is not consuming only certain types of food. It is a pathway to an ideal **sustainable weight for a lifetime.**

Photo History

Over a period of forty years it was so easy to gain a pound or two each year and remain unmoved by it. The wake-up call came when I stood in front of the mirror that day in April with this photograph lying on the bedroom dresser.

A number of years ago I found this image in a box of old memorabilia and thought it would be entertaining to make copies for my adult children. It would be good for them to see how fit their father was in his youth. I never gave my children the photos, perhaps because I wasn't proud of being overweight. Somehow I had found it acceptable to be in shape in my youth and out of shape in my adult life. Raising a family and plunging head-long into a career had given me a "pass" on maintaining my own health.

This photograph helped inspire me to take action and return to a healthier lifestyle.

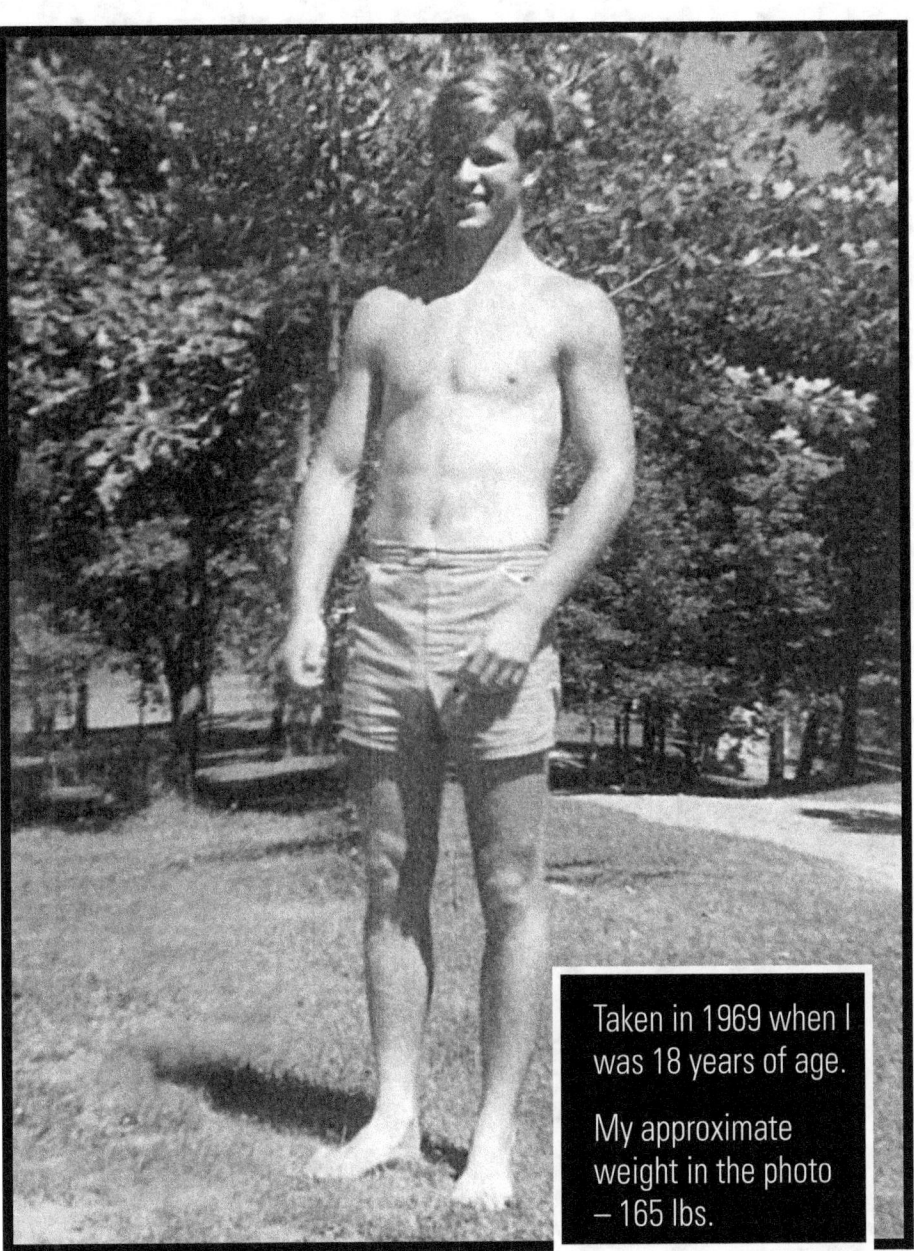

Taken in 1969 when I was 18 years of age.

My approximate weight in the photo – 165 lbs.

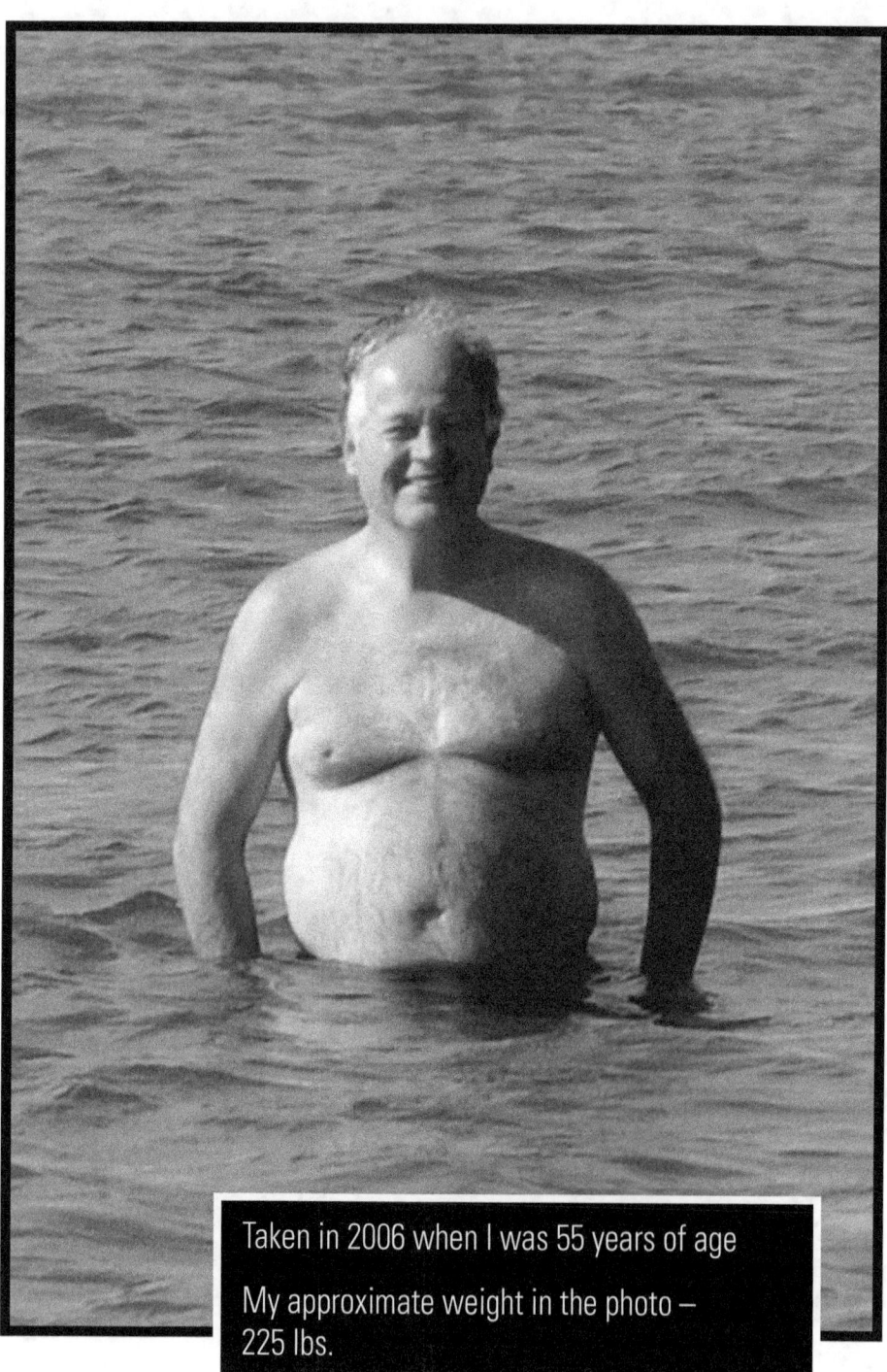

Taken in 2006 when I was 55 years of age

My approximate weight in the photo – 225 lbs.

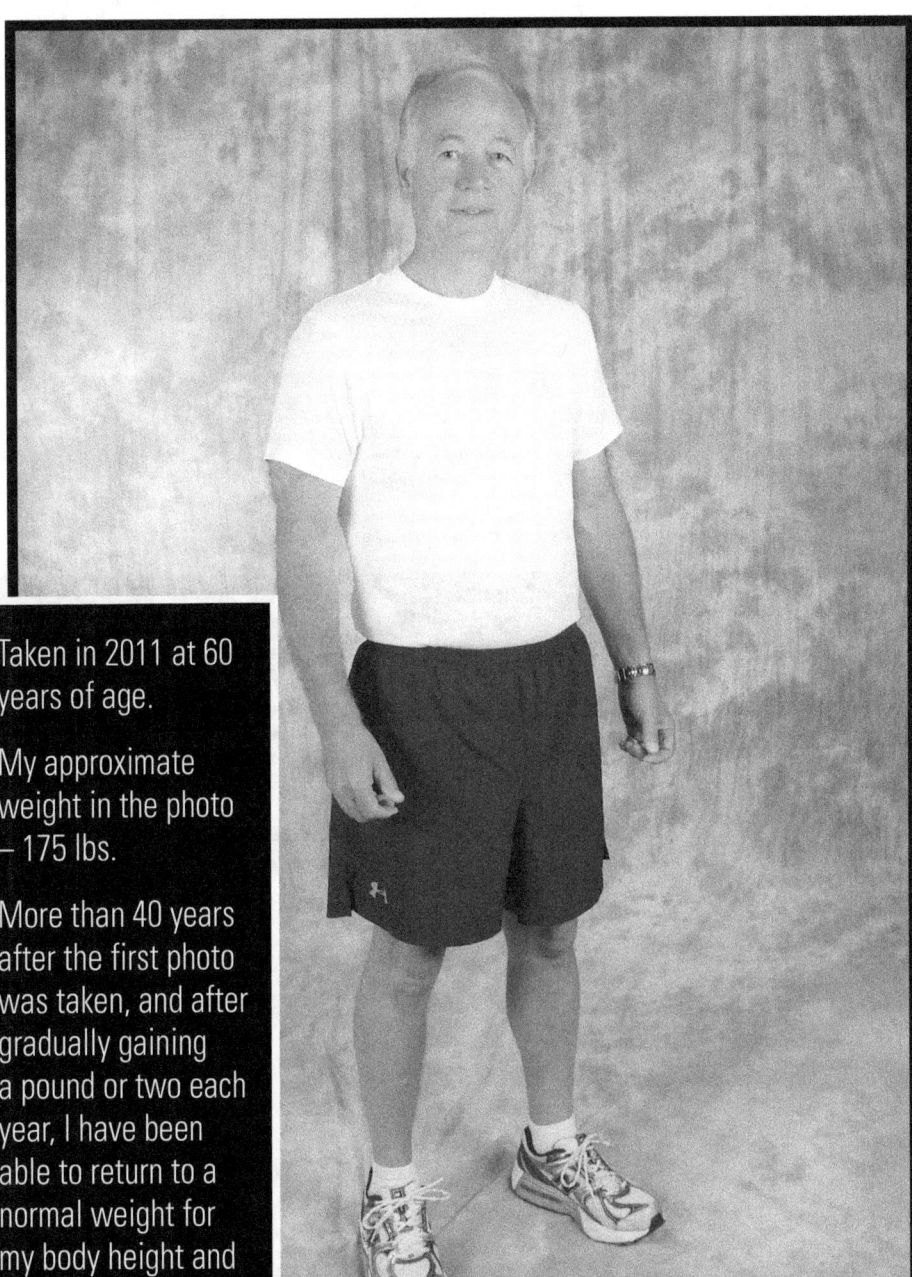

Taken in 2011 at 60 years of age.

My approximate weight in the photo – 175 lbs.

More than 40 years after the first photo was taken, and after gradually gaining a pound or two each year, I have been able to return to a normal weight for my body height and type. You can too!

As a direct result of reaching my ideal body weight, along with core strengthening exercises, at age sixty I trained for and completed a 23 Kilometer and 26 Kilometer Ski Race in Hayward, Wisconsin, on the American Birkebeiner Trail, one of the most challenging cross country ski courses in North America.

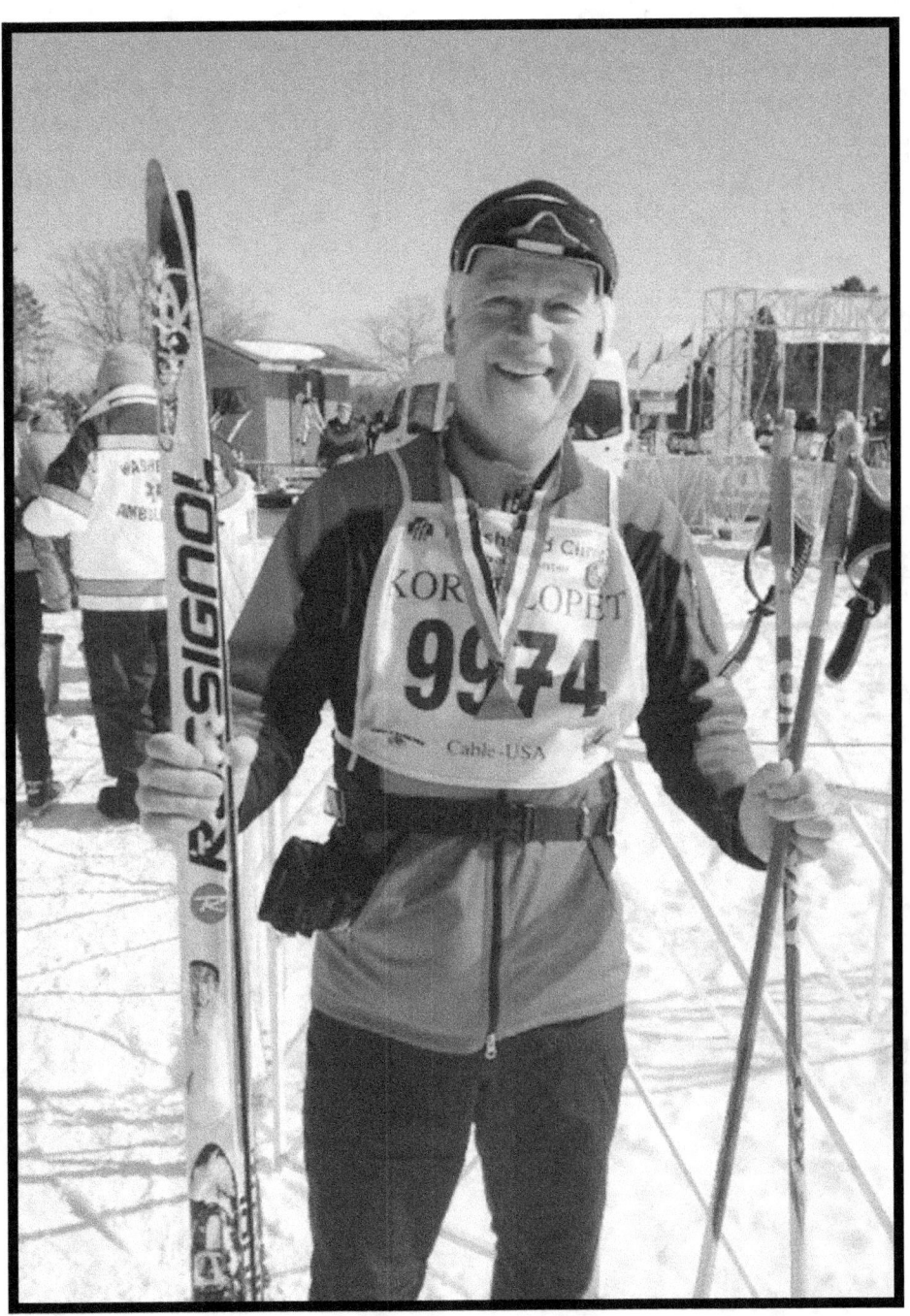

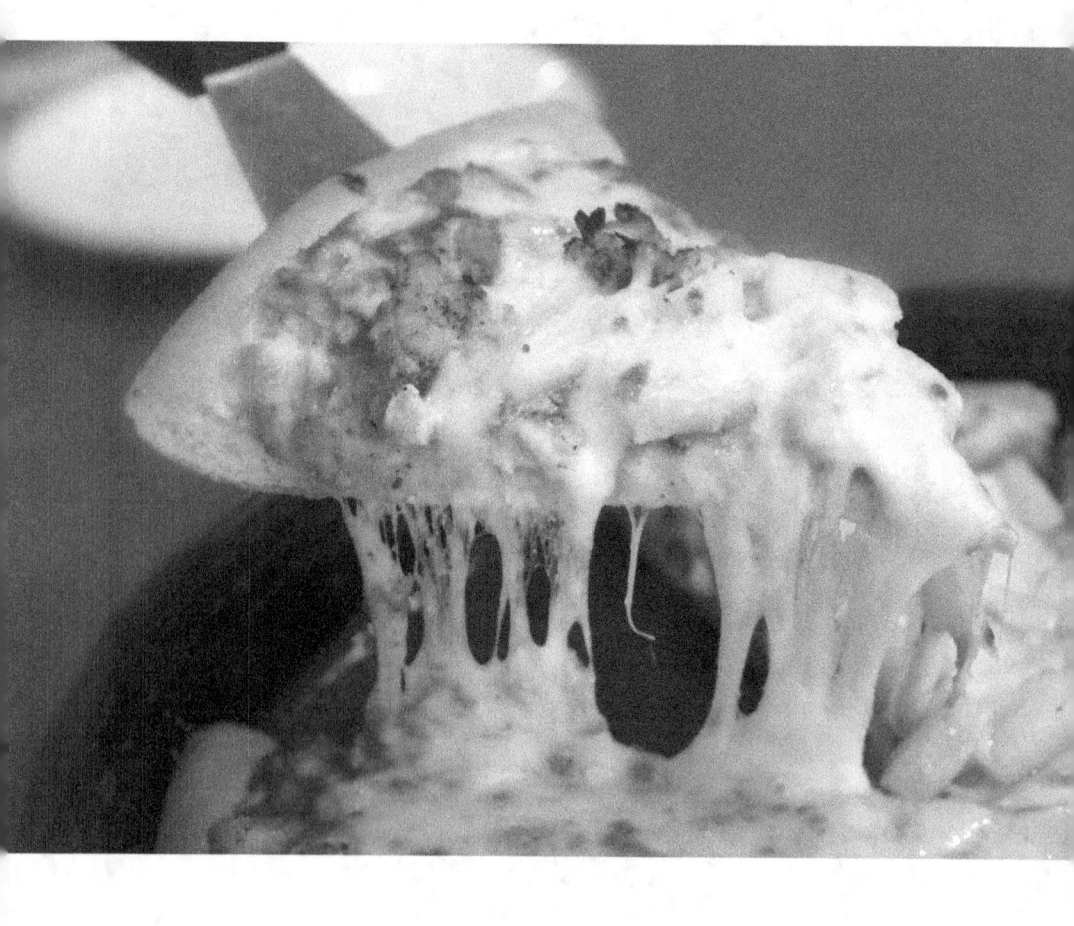

1

The world loves thin people –they just hate dieters.

I n the world of glamour, thin and fit is where it is at. Dieters, however, are inconvenient. They change the items they order at a restaurant. By special ordering they remind everyone else of the need to stay fit right in the midst of ordering a pizza. Try asking the server to hold the sour cream or go with no butter on an English muffin or light on the cheese with your pizza, and you quickly become the antagonist at the table. The trick is to order those adjustments quickly and with confidence. Be prepared with your order and its fine tuning before the server even arrives. When placing your order at a restaurant, it is essential to remember the staff is there to take care of you-not the other way around. Do not be pressured by the server to shorten up your order or feel that customizing your order is somehow out of line—it is not. Omit certain toppings and ask for others on the side so you can control the portion size. If you get a negative response from the waiter, smile and be persistent. Your health overrules the waiter's time and effort.

Recently when visiting my parents at their winter retreat on the gulf coast, we went out for beignets, a southern pastry. In a group of six, I indicated I only wanted one whereas everyone else ordered two. After I ordered, my mother spoke up and said, "You were more fun when you weren't dieting." This is the same mother who had encouraged me to lose weight for years. Overcome the fear of rejection, and you can eat what *you* want and be on your way to healthier living.

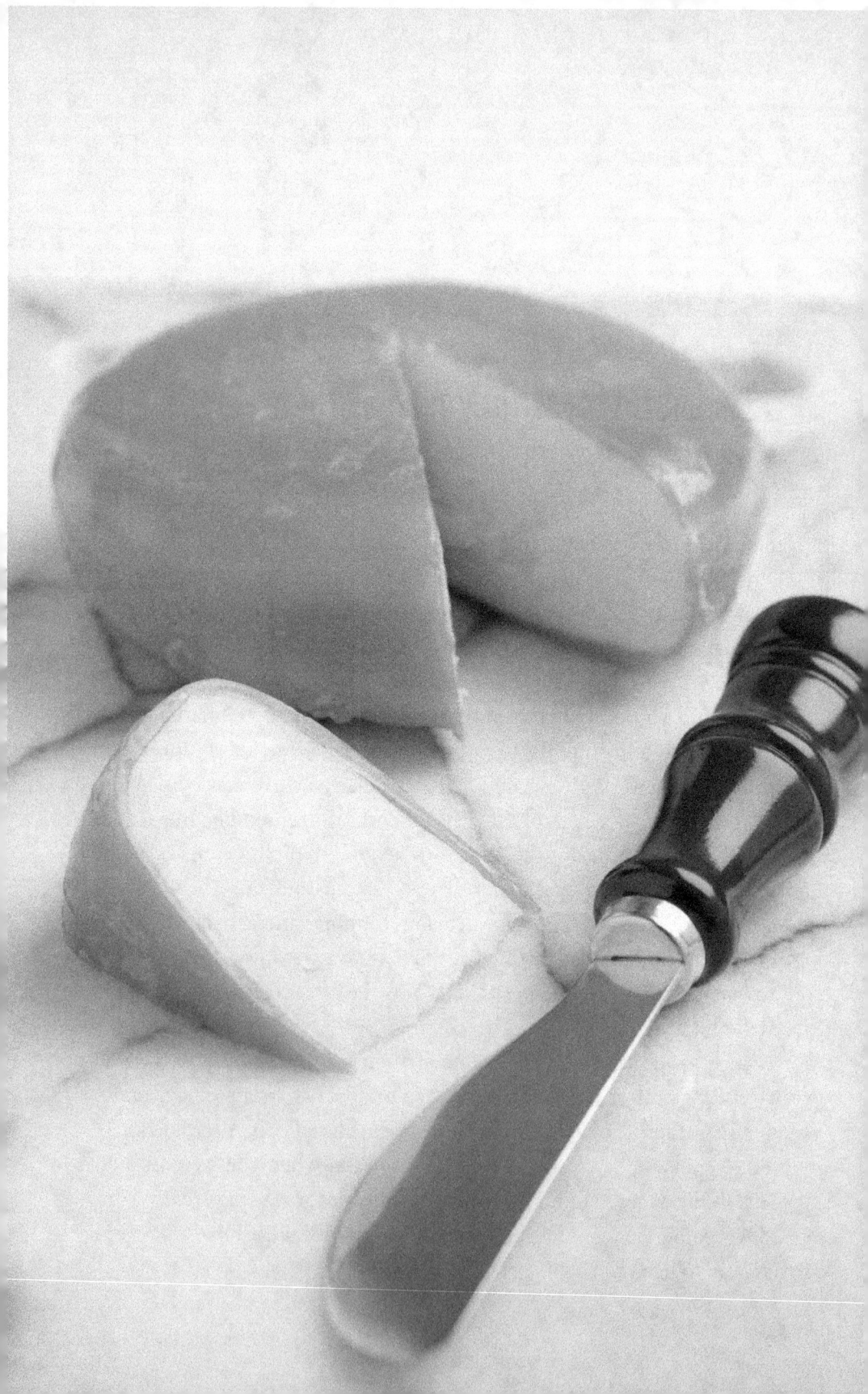

2

Divide and conquer.

Ever sit home at night reading a book or watching television and get a craving to eat something? Probably. Is this normal? Probably. How do you handle this urge? The best way is by the Divide and Conquer Principle. If you go to the refrigerator and look at an apple that you bought to make your refrigerator look healthy, you may move on to something less healthy. If, however, you take the apple out of the refrigerator and slice it into eight wedges, it is amazing how good it tastes. If you look at a block of your favorite cheese in your refrigerator, and place it on a plate with a side of buttery crackers, you will satisfy your hunger and hate yourself when you get on the treadmill in the morning. Undoubtedly you will slice away throughout the night, and, before you know it, most of the cheese is gone. Try taking the cheese from the refrigerator and cutting off a small section. Then cut that section into six to eight smaller pieces. Add healthy crackers and a tall glass of cold water, and you are on your way to enjoying the night and loving yourself in the morning. The timeless saying "the idle mind is the devil's workshop" aptly applies to the consumption of food. During the day when you are active with work or other activities, those activities are a distraction to eating food. At night while curled up on the couch watching television or reading a book, the food monster is ever present. It is easy to become bored after supper and foods like hot buttered popcorn and potato chips can quickly cancel out burned calories from your work or exercise earlier that day. Losing weight will not be a painless process. You will need to remind yourself about the physical impact excess weight has on your body and your life. That reminder will help you manage weak moments at the end of your day.

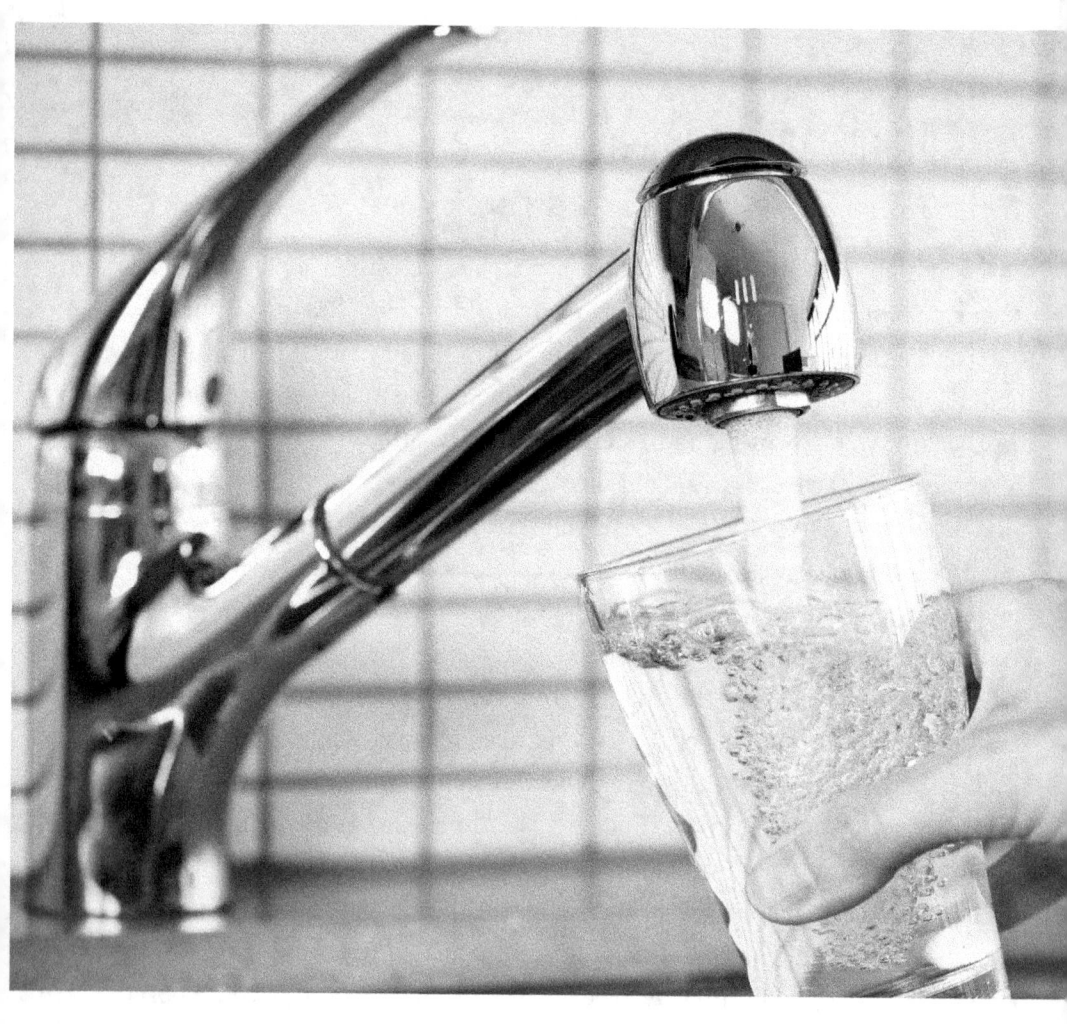

3

Water, water everywhere and not a drop to drink.

The *Rime of the Ancient Mariner* took place in the middle of an ocean. You, on the other hand, have no excuse. Your house has good water everywhere. You can fill your stomach with twelve ounces of cold water or twelve ounces of chips and dip. The latter makes a great first impression but will come back to bite you in the butt every time. Since weight loss involves exercise, keeping your fluid intake up is essential for a healthy body. To take it a step further, add electrolytes to your water which will enhance your workout and enhance absorption of critical ions into your bloodstream such as sodium, potassium and calcium. These electrolytes positively affect and regulate hydration, restore blood pH, and improve nerve and muscular functionality, both during and after a good workout. Electrolytes are easily available for purchase or included in a variety of beverages. I keep a thirty-two ounce water bottle with me in the gym and at my desk. It is amazing how refreshed you feel after a swallow or two. Water is the source of all life, and you are no exception. So go ahead and indulge yourself in lots of water every day.

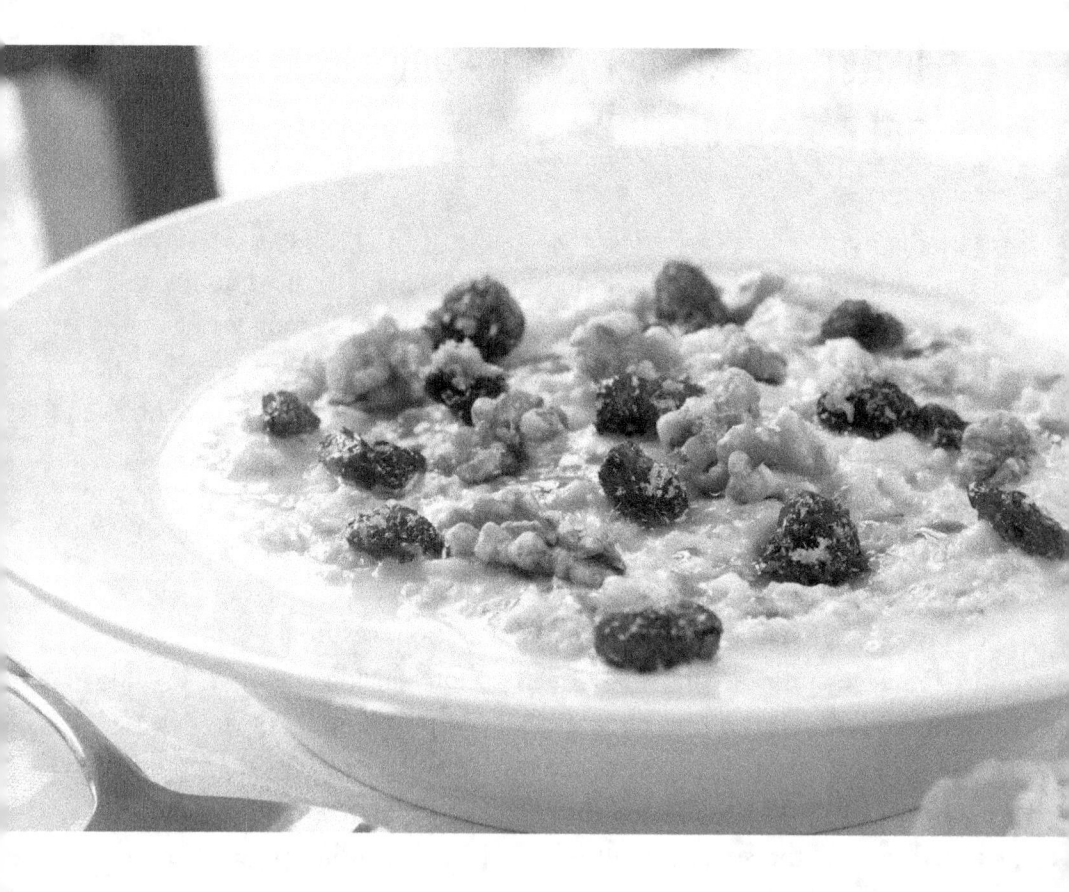

4

Fire up your engine.

You have heard it from everyone—breakfast is the most important meal of the day. So why do so many people skip that meal? We have to go to work, we have no time to eat, and we can grab a cup of coffee at work. At work there are also sweet rolls and brownies, which, by the time you get there, sound too good to pass up since your stomach just started growling. Who has time for breakfast when you have a client waiting in your office or you have to be punched in at 8:00 a.m.? You do have time for a grain or bran cereal and a beverage – even fruit. Our society has ingrained in us the breakfast staple of bacon, eggs, toast, and beverage—even hash browns—and all prepared in what? Yes, grease and butter. Oatmeal doesn't sound very glamorous, but try it with fresh berries or a mixture of raisins and dates on top, and you are on your way to a great day. These are sure ways to fire up your system, and it's even good for you!

Another important way to start your morning is with a protein shake. No, not the kind you buy in a can in the store, but a homemade shake that literally takes three minutes to make and tastes so good you will forget you are on a weight-loss program. Go to the store and purchase a couple of bags of frozen fruit, then pick up whey protein at your closest nutritional food outlet. Purchase a mini-blender for a nominal amount of money, and you are ready to begin your day with breakfast. Whey protein helps build muscle and prevents muscle wasting and it comes in multiple flavors. Just add water, whey, and fruit to the blender, mix, pour, and drink. You can mix it up with bananas, peanut butter, mandarin oranges, or whatever you like. Add a side of oatmeal or healthy grain cereal, and its Hi Ho, Hi Ho, and off to work you go!

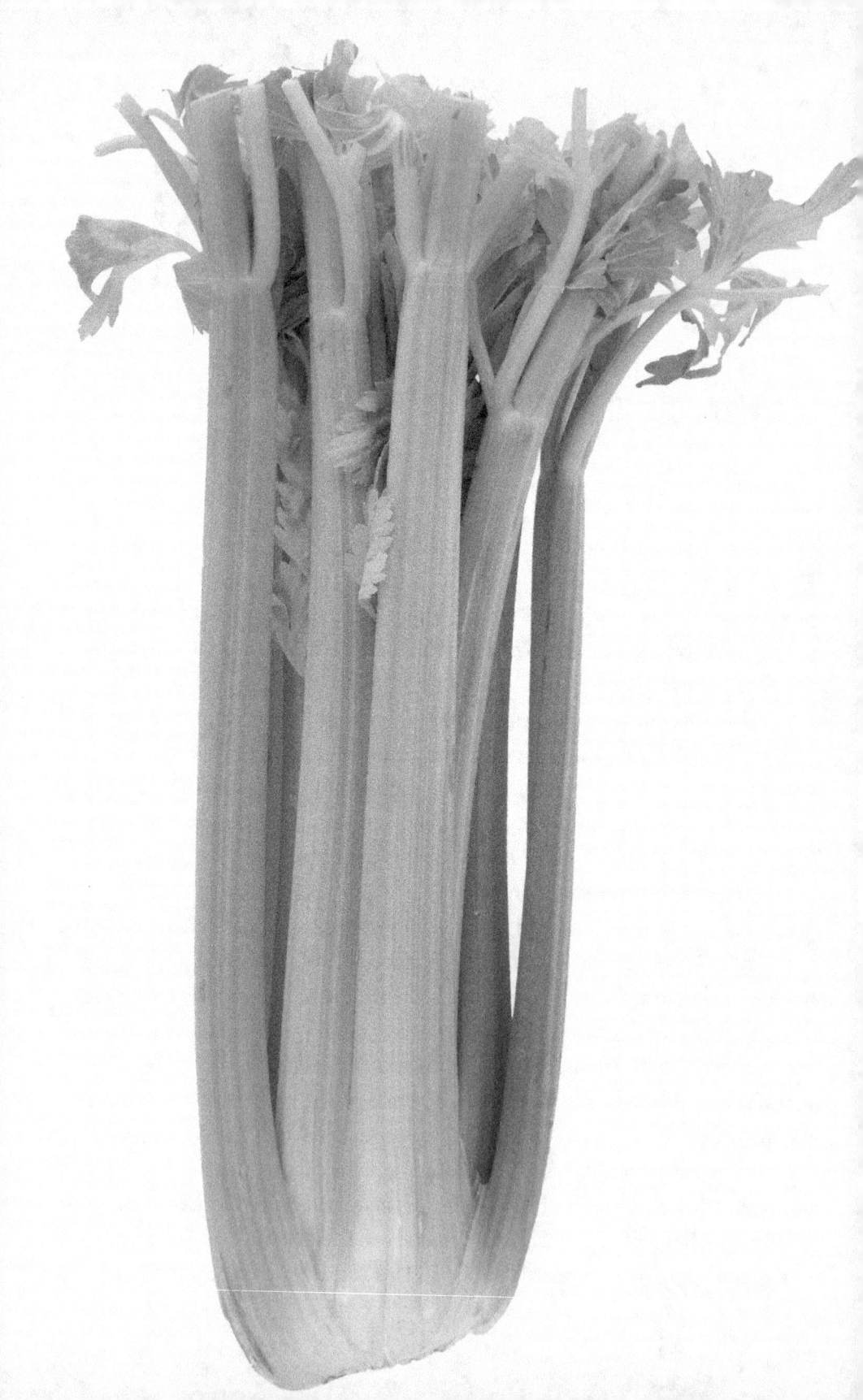

5

Avoid the word "diet."

You will notice that other than in chapter 1 and 5, this four-letter word has been deliberately omitted from the entire book. That is because people hate dieting. When talking about weight control, this word is one of the most over used words in the English language. It elicits painful images of hard work and eating celery. To accomplish your goal of losing weight, never use the word diet. Instead it is a lifestyle change of healthy eating and exercise. Try to understand that the only way to accomplish your goal is to not deny yourself any of the things you like to eat—just the quantity and frequency. The words to remember are "sustainable weight loss." Why punish yourself? Who would ever stay on any program for a lifetime if every day was a painful experience? And yet almost every available weight-loss program involves trying to train or trick your body to do something it just doesn't want to do. How long can you stay on this type of weight loss program? One month? Six months? A year? What good is that when you are planning to live for decades? The protein-only diets, the liquid diets, and the nationally televised diets all have one thing in common: they are unsustainable, and that is why they fail.

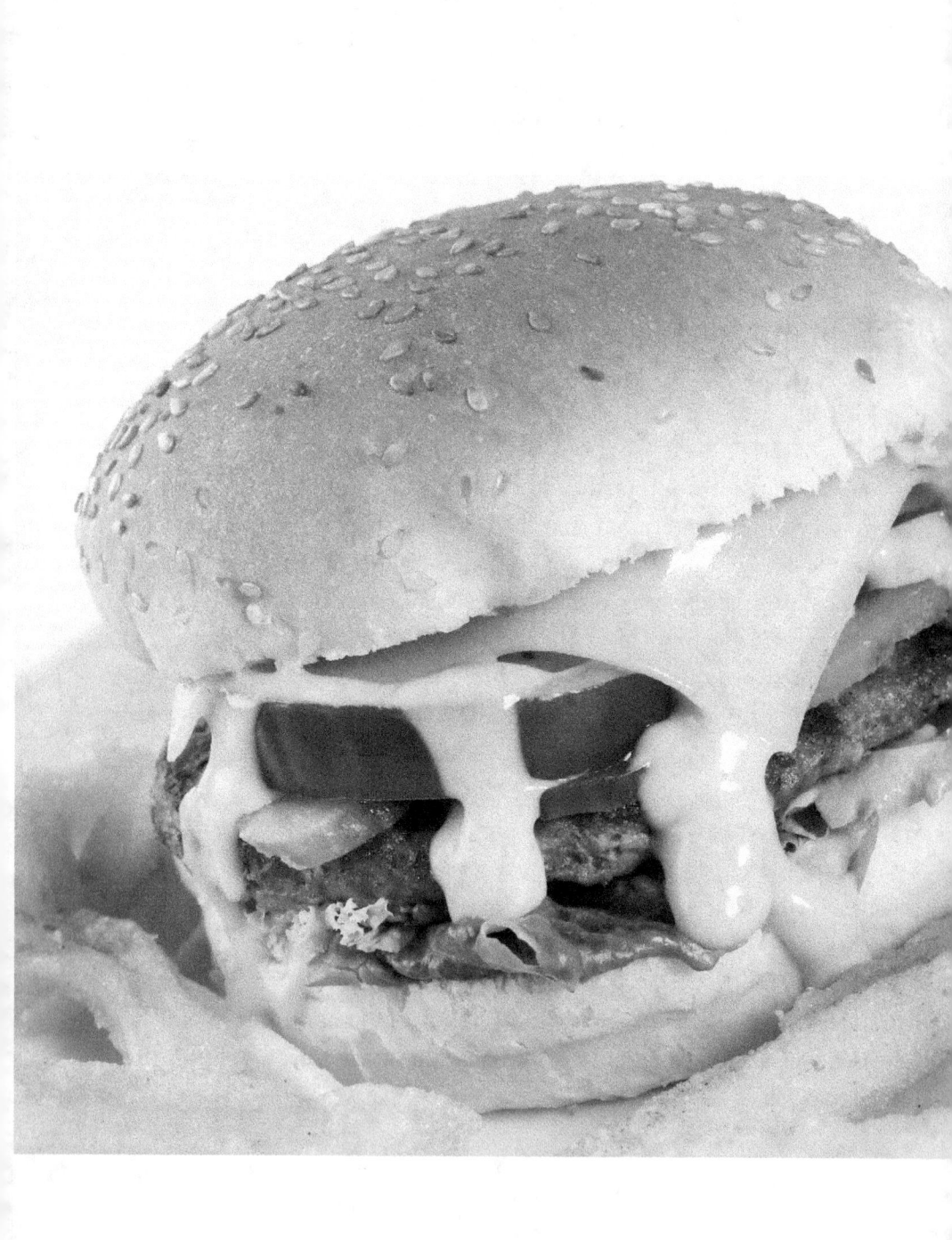

6

Plain as the nose on your face.

ong before I started to change the quantity and the quality of food I ate, I began to think of food in a more simplistic way. I stopped putting grilled onions and ketchup on my hamburgers, stopped drowning my potato in butter and sour cream, and stopped putting unhealthy toppings on all my foods. What I discovered was that a grilled hamburger actually tasted better without all the extras. Potatoes and other vegetables actually had unique flavors of their own; I always thought they tasted like sour cream and butter. Using any of these items once in a while is not a problem, but daily or at every meal the calories quickly add up, and so does the buildup on your waistline and the walls of your arteries.

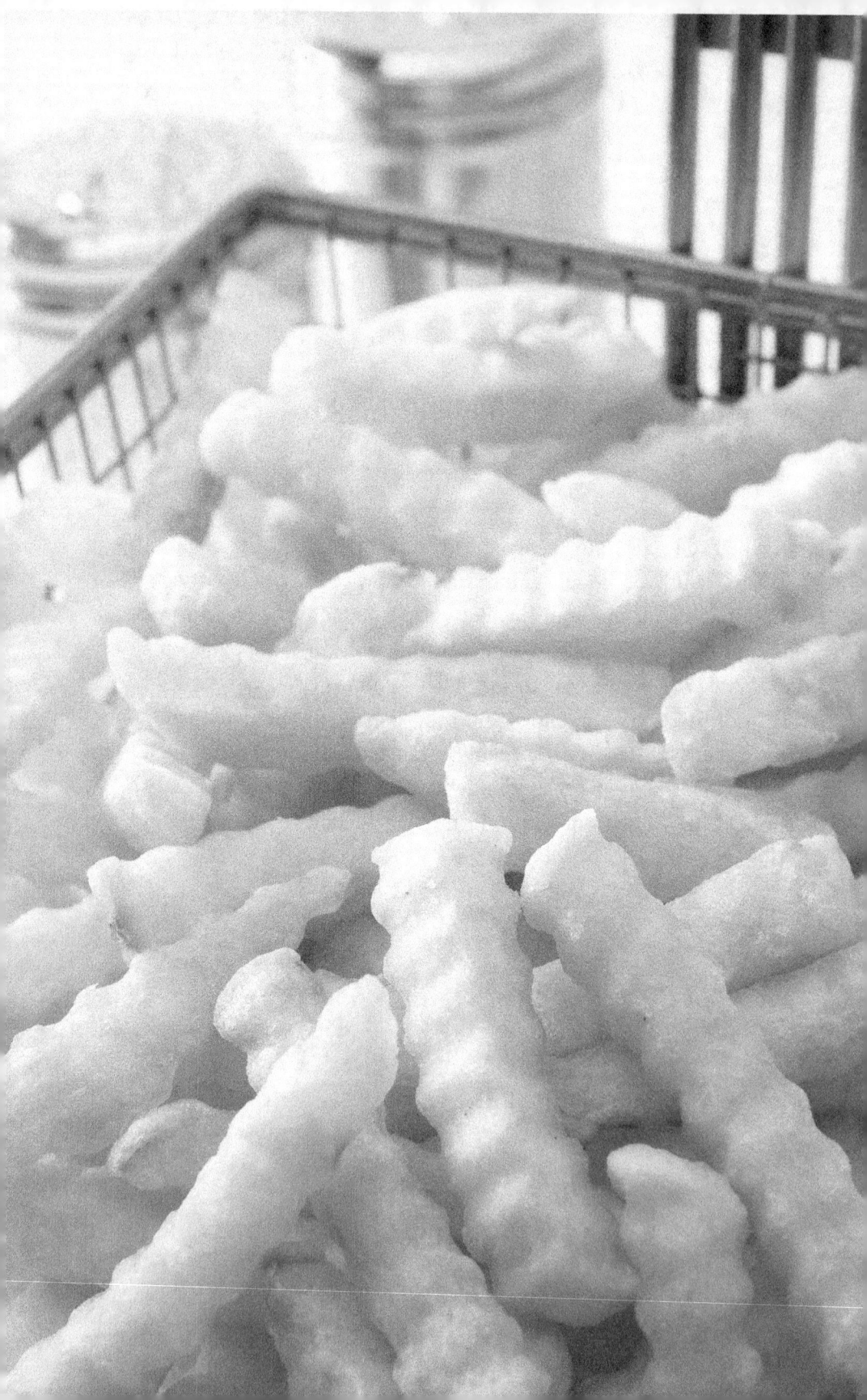

7

Grease is not the word.

Contrary to the movie, grease is the one item in the American diet that you must do without. Will an occasional French fry or order of onion rings hurt you? No, I still eat those foods—just not often. Up until recently, my cholesterol was high, and I had been on a medication to correct it for years. Once I lost weight and stopped eating fried foods, not only did my cholesterol drop to where I could rid myself of the medication but my test results place me in the upper 10th percentile for the right cholesterol nationwide. These medications are used prolifically in the United States. You cannot turn on a television without seeing an ad for one variety or another. While they assist in lowering cholesterol, they also are very hard on your liver and other organs you can't live without. In more recent years, restaurants have turned to a more vegetable based grease, but in the end it is still way too much.

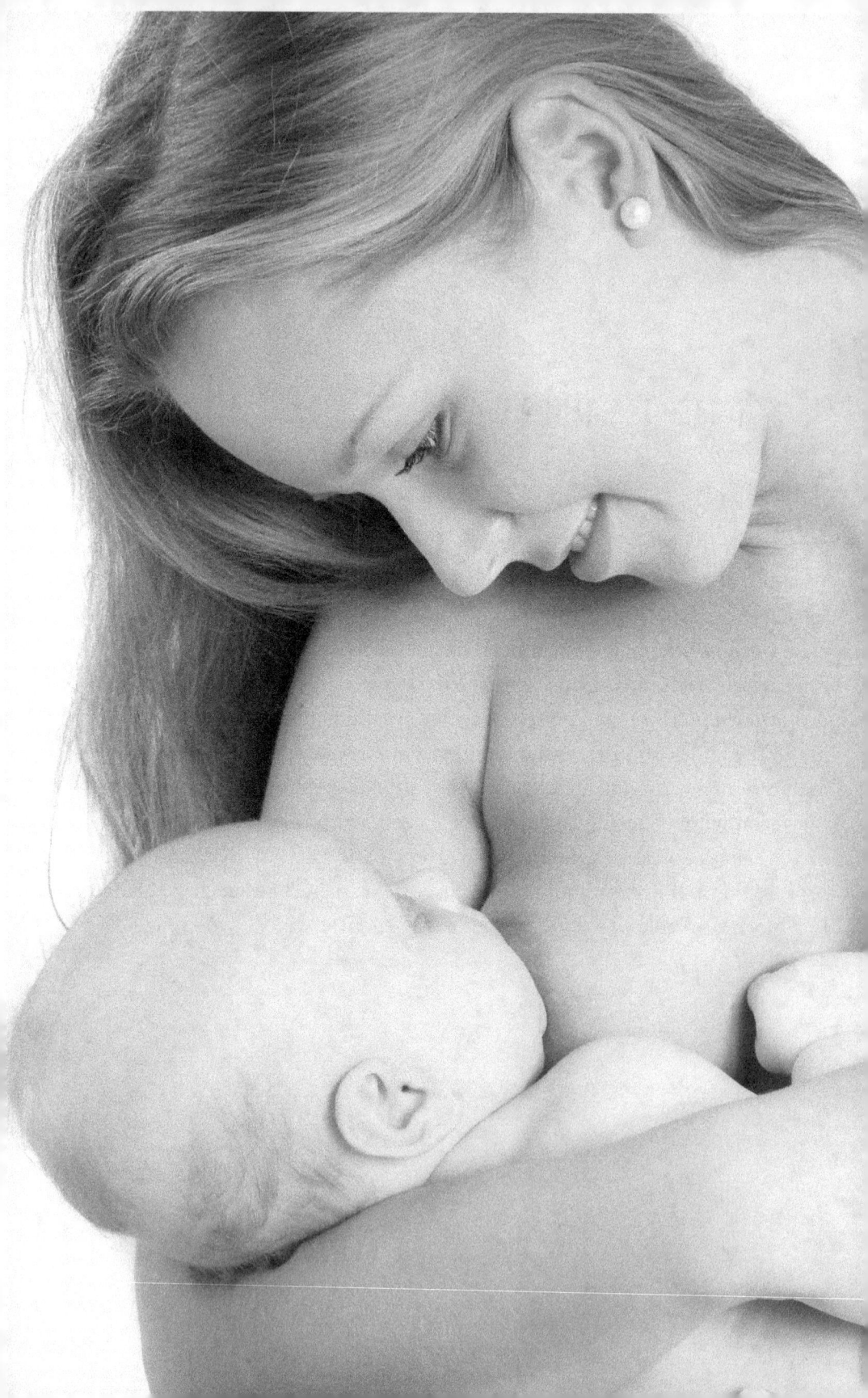

8

All things in moderation.

We have all heard the above phrase for years. It can be true, but it can also give us an excuse to drift from our true goal—sustainable weight loss. How do we gauge moderation? Moderation to one individual is excess to another. That said it is not a good idea to say, "I will never eat that again." Denying yourself the foods you love creates an impediment to your goal and makes you angry about having to lose weight. So go ahead and eat chocolate cake or chips and dip on occasion. It is OK to occasionally reward yourself for justifiable progress. After all, you are the best coach for your own body.

What about how we eat? Years ago I worked with a man who lived on fast food for lunch. A stop at his favorite hamburger place would yield two extra-large hamburgers, an extra-large French fry, and a large chocolate shake. I would be part way through my hamburger when I observed him putting his two large hamburger wrappings back in the bag. The sheer volume of calories and fat intake was one thing, but the speed at which he devoured the food was amazing. This illustration brings me to my point: take small bites. Naturally, we are born with an oral fixation that begins at birth with a mother nursing her child and then is manifested throughout life as we eat food and drink beverages. Beyond the nutritional need we have for eating is the need to satisfy the urge to put something in our mouth. Consider how unsatisfied the man in my last example must have been. While the food filled his stomach, it did not satisfy his need for oral satisfaction and consequently he continued to eat other foods throughout the day. Enjoy the food you eat with smaller bite sizes. Make your mealtime a more satisfying experience by extending its duration. Your body will thank you for it.

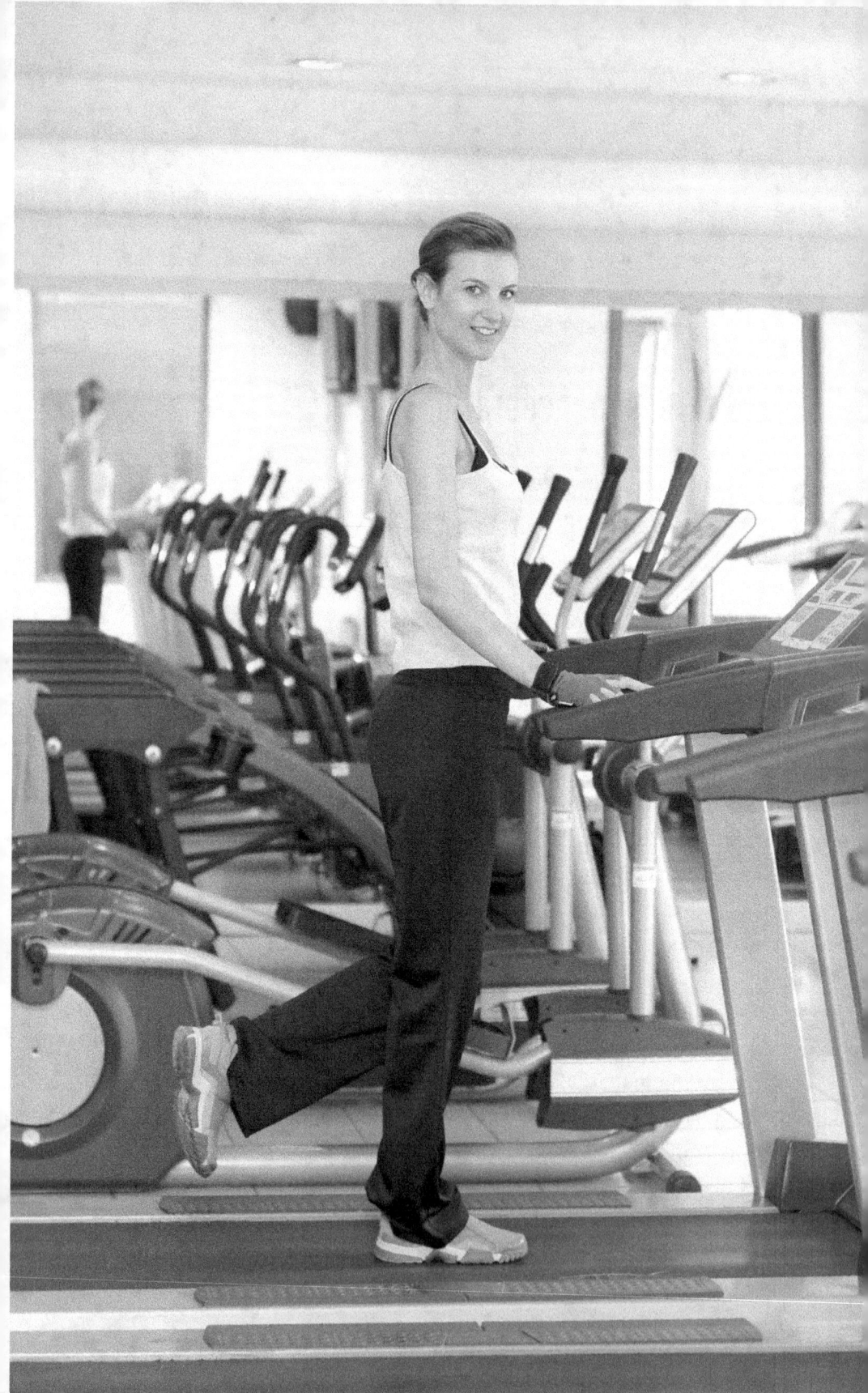

9

Run to win.

The best companion to proper eating is exercise. This word conjures up all sorts of images including pain, sweat, and early morning wake up calls. Nevertheless, once you make the commitment to exercise, you will appreciate the great emotional lift to your day, especially after your post workout shower, and never return to your old lifestyle. There are volumes of books and workout manuals devoted to instructing you on the right pathway for success. In my opinion, the best pathway to success is the power treadmill. And why not? Walking and running are natural movements our bodies know and understand. For diversity you can auto-adjust speeds or create inclines. You can even add to the experience by working with three-pound hand weights. Elliptical machines and stair-climbers are good, but I do not believe they are sustainable for a lifetime. They can, however, add diversity to your workout as you later transition to "in the gym" workouts.

As you get closer to your ideal body weight, add weight training to your regimen. For me this happened about one year after I began my program for sustainable weight loss. Building and toning muscles is another essential ingredient for a healthy body. Muscle supports the structural integrity of your body–bones. Consider hiring a personal trainer for one hour per week to get you off on the right program. Pulling a muscle or injuring your back through poor body mechanics will not only slow your progress but could cause a long-term injury. A few simple guidelines for muscle toning are as follows: Exercise early in the day before you go to work. This will allow your body to start burning calories early. After a workout your body will continue to burn calories for another few hours. People who workout at lunchtime or after supper miss this opportunity. A side benefit is the refreshed and revitalized person that you will become as you head into your work day. I always thought an early workout would make me tired and too weak to attack the work day—just the opposite is true. And, believe it or not, the early workout sessions become something you look forward to - with the added bonus of an early start to your day.

Next, toning your muscles involves all segments of your body—legs, abdominals, and upper torso. As part of your workout routine, alternate weight training and cardio sessions to avoid stressing your body, but always do a brief fifteen minute cardio session prior to the weights. This short session gets your blood and heart pumping for a more effective workout. When working on weights there are three key phrases to remember: "slow and in control," "pace the weights," and "listen to your body." It is easy to get started with early energy and want to move through the exercises quickly. Working your muscles slowly, while controlling your body movement, will ensure a safe and thorough workout. When adding weight to each workout, remember to pace your changes—start with smaller weights and increase incrementally as the weeks go by. You can bump up the weight a small amount on the second round of your routine if you are ready for it. Your goal is not to enter a body building competition; it is to create a healthy lifestyle. Above all, listen to your body. If you don't, injuries will occur.

Recently, while going through my weight training routine, I had a pre-exercise meeting with my trainer on safety—how toning was the most important element in the exercise process, not "body-building." I wanted to eliminate one of the exercises because it felt like it was putting disproportionate stress on my lower back. I decided not to mention it, and later that day I sustained a minor injury to my lower back that kept me out of the fitness center for a few days while I rested, applied ice and went around the clock with anti-inflammatory medication. Remember these exercise essentials: "slow and in control," "pace the weights," and "listen to your body" to extend your lifetime many years into the future. (See Appendix A for my workout regimens)

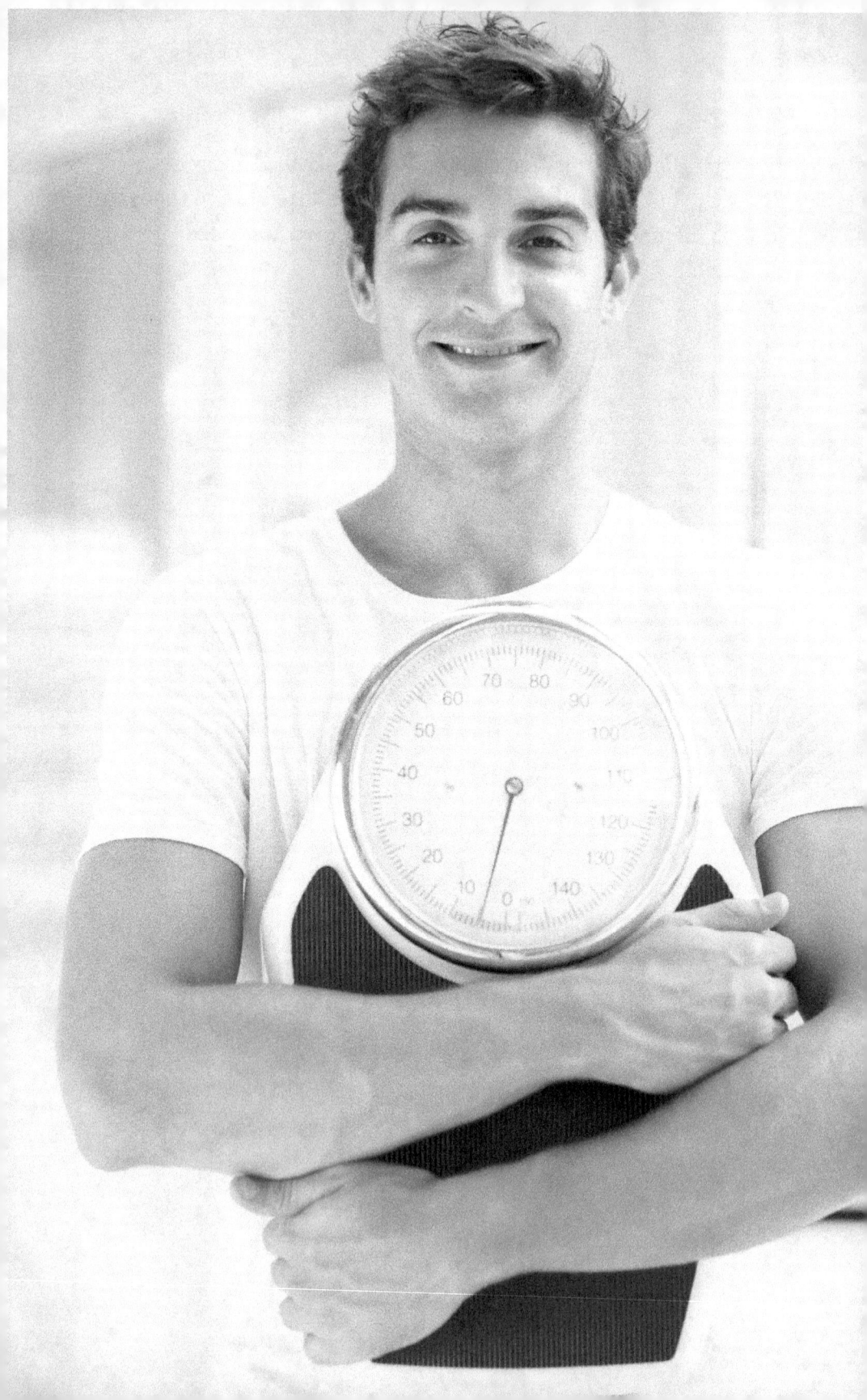

10

Slow cook.

Whenever we decide it is time to do something, there is a strong tendency to want to accomplish the task all at once. We want it when we want it, and we want it our way. We are a "fast food society." Transition out of this type of world and embrace a slower, more rewarding pace to reach an ideal body weight. Remember, it didn't take you a month to reach your current weight—it took years. The process to remove it will take time as well, and hurrying it along will only add frustration to the process. Once frustrated, quitting is not far behind. Cherish each step on the way to success. Excess weight took a long time to become part of your body so don't be disheartened when progress is slow. Even two pounds a month is twenty-four pounds in one year so don't try to accomplish this change in three months. Quick weight loss equals quick weight gain after you tire of the process.

Have you ever talked with someone who was on a liquid diet? How did they look a year or two later? In most cases they were back to their old weight and in many cases heavier. Is it possible to sustain a liquid diet for a lifetime? No, it is not. A well-planned, long-term program is the only way to effectively lose weight and maintain a healthy weight for a lifetime.

Charting your weight change is important but only weigh once a week. Daily tracking will only serve to create uncertainty and potentially be an impediment to your progress. Because eating habits are changing, you will plateau at times and maybe even bump up a pound or two. This is completely natural, but it is also when most people stop trying. Your body is just adjusting to your changes and building muscle. If you stay the course, you will break through that plateau and move forward to your target weight. To reach your target weight, this cycle will be repeated multiple times. (See Appendix B for my personal weight chart)

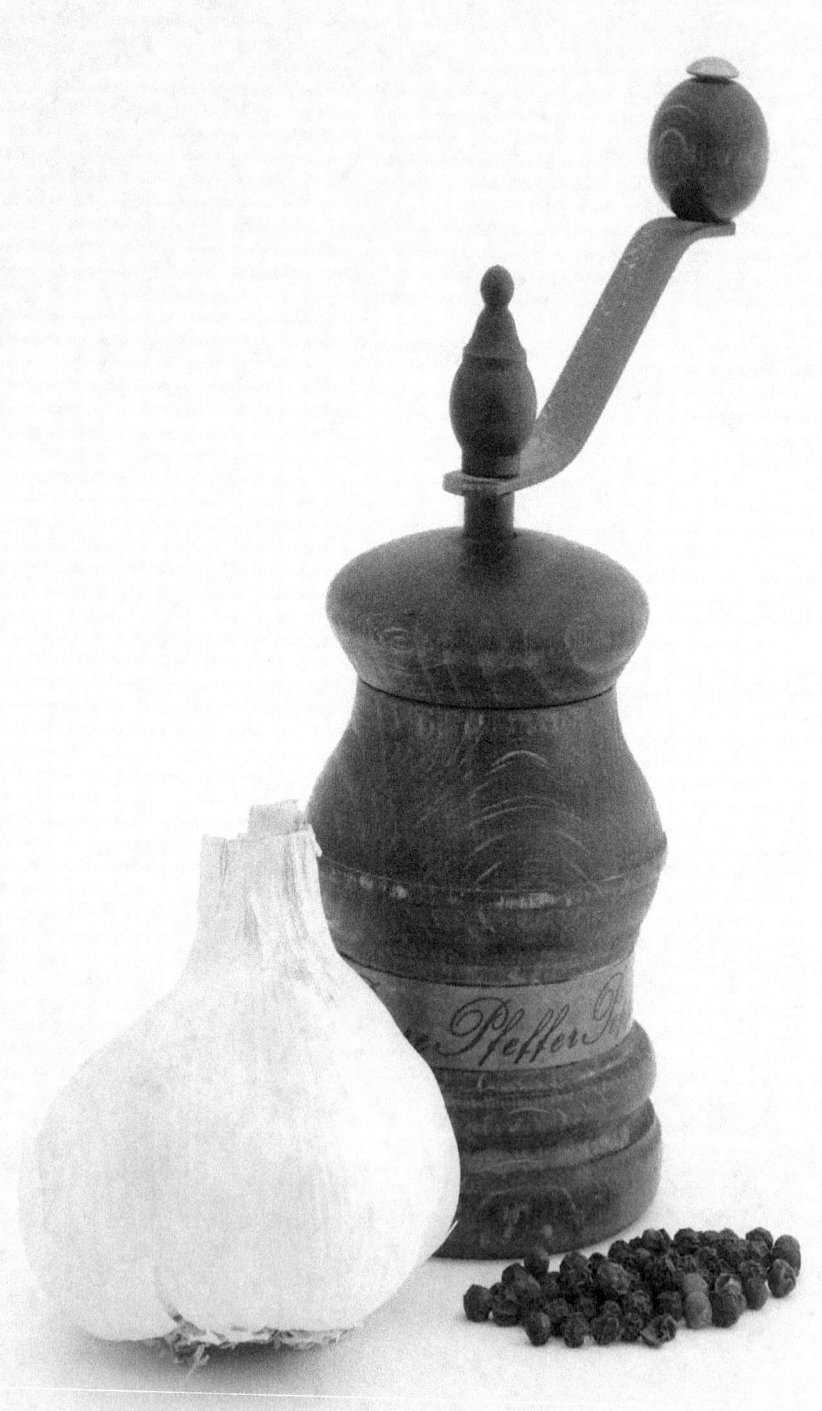

11

Taste the food with smart flavorings.

How many spices and other toppings do you have in your kitchen? Undoubtedly dozens. Then why do we only use six of them? Many of us drown our food in salt, ketchup, mustard, heavy dressings, sour cream, or cheese. You may have a different list. What about rosemary, basil, balsamic vinegar, chopped garlic, cinnamon, or fresh-ground pepper? There are many more. The second group can flavor the food we eat, add healthy properties to our body, and cut unnecessary calorie intake.

While touring Italy this past year, my wife and I dined out many times. Wherever we dined there was a stark contrast to the American restaurant. First, the portion sizes were smaller—not super-sized—and buffets did not exist. Secondly, there was no butter, cream, sugar, or salt at any table—only vinegar and olive oil. Finally, there was not a parking lot full of cars from people who drove in from the suburbs—just people walking or biking to the restaurant…imagine that. There is a common phrase in the accounting profession: "garbage in, garbage out." In the weight loss world, it is simply "garbage in, garbage stays in." Be selective with the flavorings you choose, taste the unique flavors of the food, and do not overpower food with unnecessary toppings.

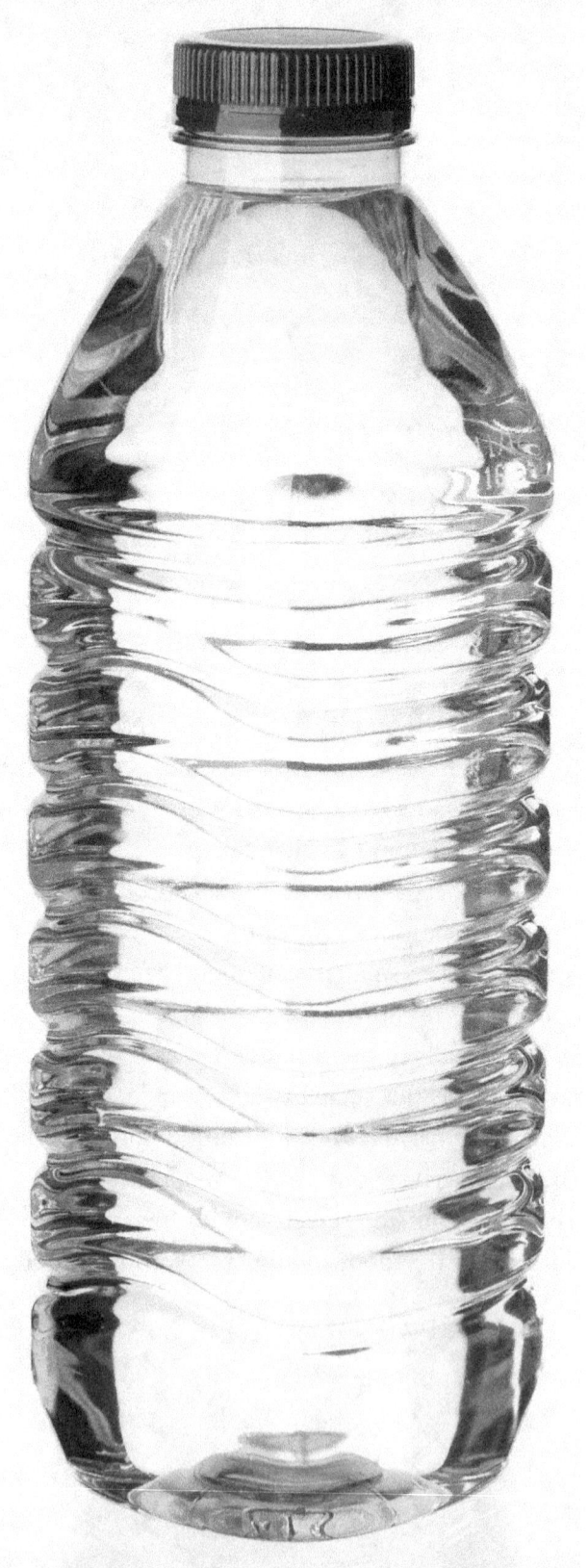

12

Can the calories.

Liquids are essential to sustain life but be selective about the liquids you add to our body. Advertisements for soda on television, radio, newspapers, internet, and billboards are contributing to obesity in America. Most of the bottled liquids in your grocer's soda aisle or cooler wall contain liquids with empty calories. Corporations have even reinvented them to make them look healthy with various vitamins and flavorings. These choices can add 150 to 250 calories to your body with each selection adding very little nutritional value. Take in three or four of these per day and you can add 1000 calories very quickly—more than a healthy dinner. And these are empty calories. A good rule to follow is to drink water for hydration and select quality liquids for taste. Rather than 1000 empty calories of soda, why not choose a vegetable drink, juice, wine, milk, or even a robust tap beer? With these selections you are getting great flavor and important nutrition in your selection.

To take it a step further, sugar is a poor nutritional element and it is everywhere – soda, baked goods, cereals and candy products. Sugar adds empty calories to your body while giving a temporary boost in energy. On the problematic side it contributes to diabetes, osteoporosis and facilitates fat storage. Beyond sugar, another problematic element in our diet is salt. While salt is essential for maintaining normal pH in our blood, and assisting in muscular contraction - elevated levels of salt create problems with high blood pressure and heart disease. Many foods overload us with salt including processed foods, fast foods, and chips to name only a few. Recently I looked at a can of soup and was shocked to see that the two servings it contained, easily consumed by one person, represented 72% of the recommended daily allowance for salt! Get used to reading labels on the food you eat and avoid the added intake of sugar and salt.

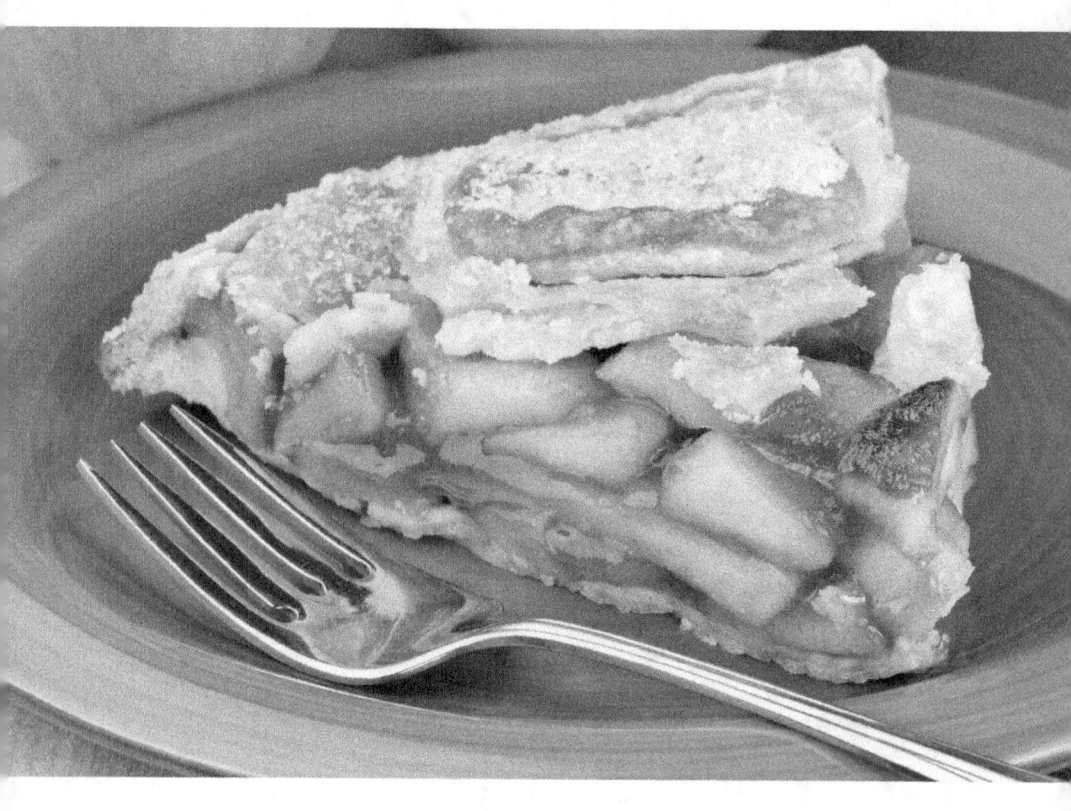

13

Choice selections.

If you choose to eat all of your favorite dishes at mealtime and in large quantities, your weight will escalate. At a holiday meal where apple pie and ice cream is the dessert, this might be the food you pass on or take home for an energy boost later that day. Keeping in the spirit of not depriving yourself of any particular food group, enjoy all the selections for the holiday–just hold down the portion size and spread out the selection. Then go for a nice long walk.

When at work the urge to eat in the late afternoon will start to nag at you, so be prepared. Don't rush out to buy a chocolate malt or a jelly donut. Have a container of dried fruit and a container of almonds at your worksite. After you pop a few, the urge to eat will dissipate, and you will be on to eating a healthy dinner later that day. While eating more meals in smaller portions throughout the day is a healthy plan, the American way of life is a three-meals-per-day routine. A little pain in the stomach while you wait until the next meal is natural, and–while popping a dried apricot mid-afternoon can be a good thing–there is always another meal ahead of you—you know the routine, breakfast, lunch, and dinner, and they cycle every day!

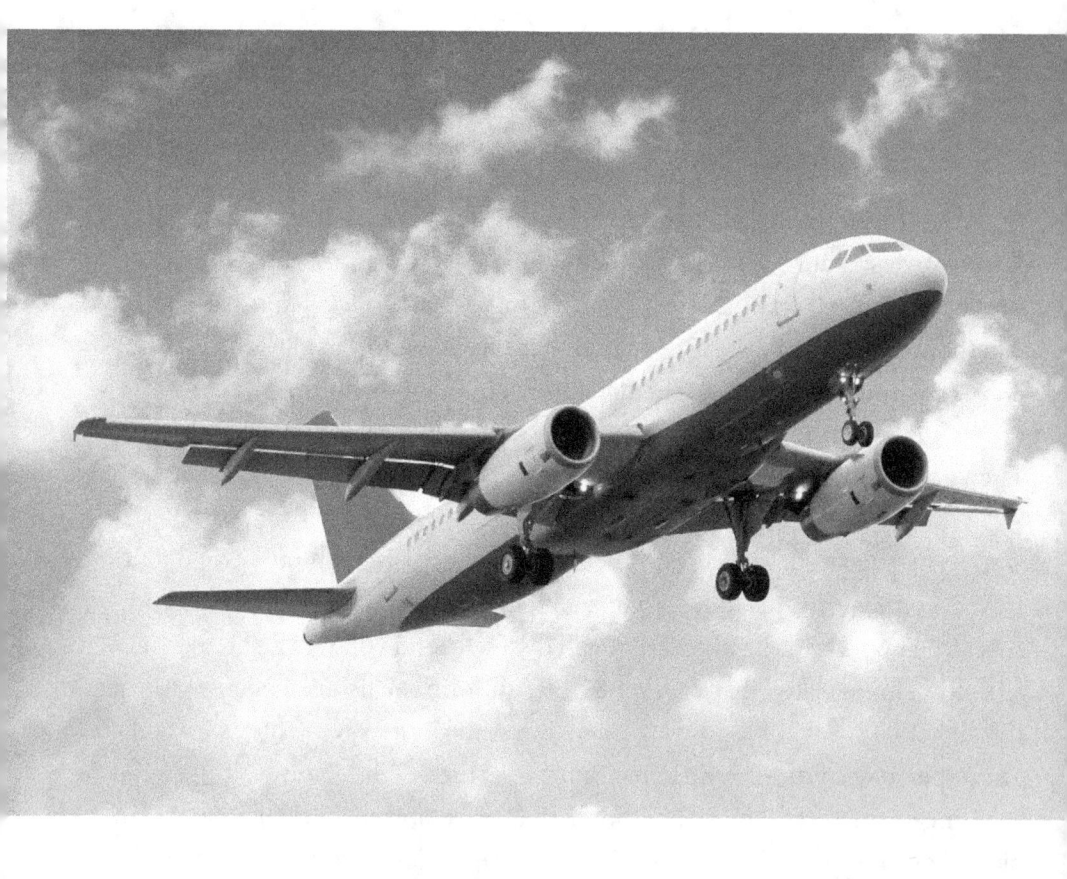

14

Lifetime companions.

In addition to eating right and getting proper exercise, there are a few additional companions to bring along for the ride:

- **Limit stress in your life** with a good night's sleep and a brief period of silence or reflection prior to beginning your day. Even as little as five minutes of reflection will help start your day with a positive mental outlook. Instead of your first conversation of the day being an intense response to a co-worker, it may be a thoughtful one.

- **Take one good multivitamin** with a high dose of vitamin D per day as directed by your physician. Yes, some of the vitamins might flush out of your system due to higher doses than needed, but others will supply you with nutrients you fell short on that day. Avoid heavy-duty supplements–nothing replaces the real thing in your body!

- **Maintain good oral hygiene.** Several years ago I was on the verge of periodontal disease, not because I didn't brush my teeth, but because I did not floss or use a tongue blade. With the recommendations of friends, I sought out a new dentist, and within six months I was able to reverse the problems and symptoms I was experiencing.

Your selection of a dentist is of equal importance to your selection of a physician.

- **Take a vacation and days off just for you.** The phrase "all work and no play make Jack a dull boy" is true in many ways. You will find that time off is an essential ingredient to a successful lifestyle. No time off equals burnout, and that will affect your weight. Time off will reenergize your mind and body and allow you to effectively navigate through your life.

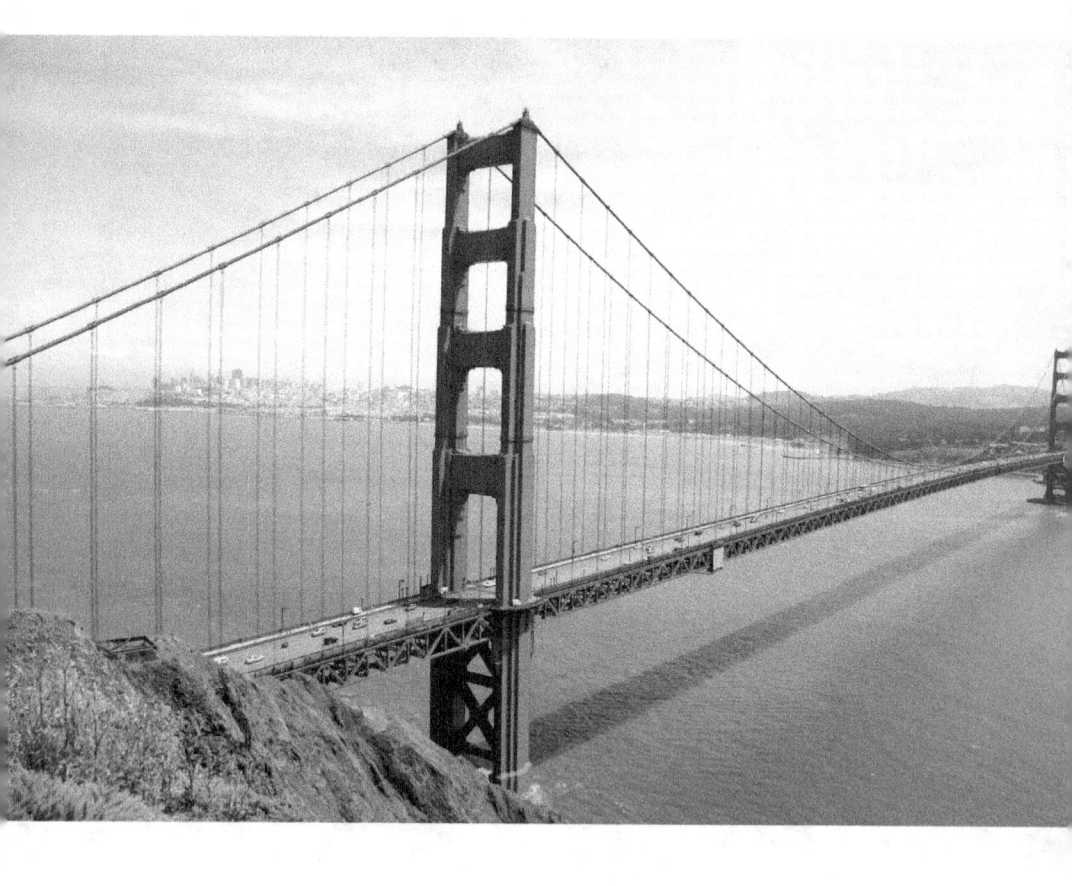

15

Crossing over.

I n this case I am not referring to a near-death experience but to the point in time when your body no longer needs the heavy duty coaxing to eat healthy. It is when you no longer *push* to eat healthy but when your body *demands* to eat healthy. The urge to eat a double cheeseburger is now substituted with the desire to eat sautéed or steamed vegetables or a turkey sandwich.

Crossing over is also the time when your body rejects certain foods. My favorite fish dinner can still be enjoyed as long as I order baked or perhaps pan fried. A full dinner of deep fried fish will no longer set well in my stomach, and I no longer have the desire to order it. In my case, the crossing over milestone took one year to reach. Yours will undoubtedly be a different timetable. This is the day you have been waiting for—to no longer struggle to be at a sustainable weight for a lifetime.

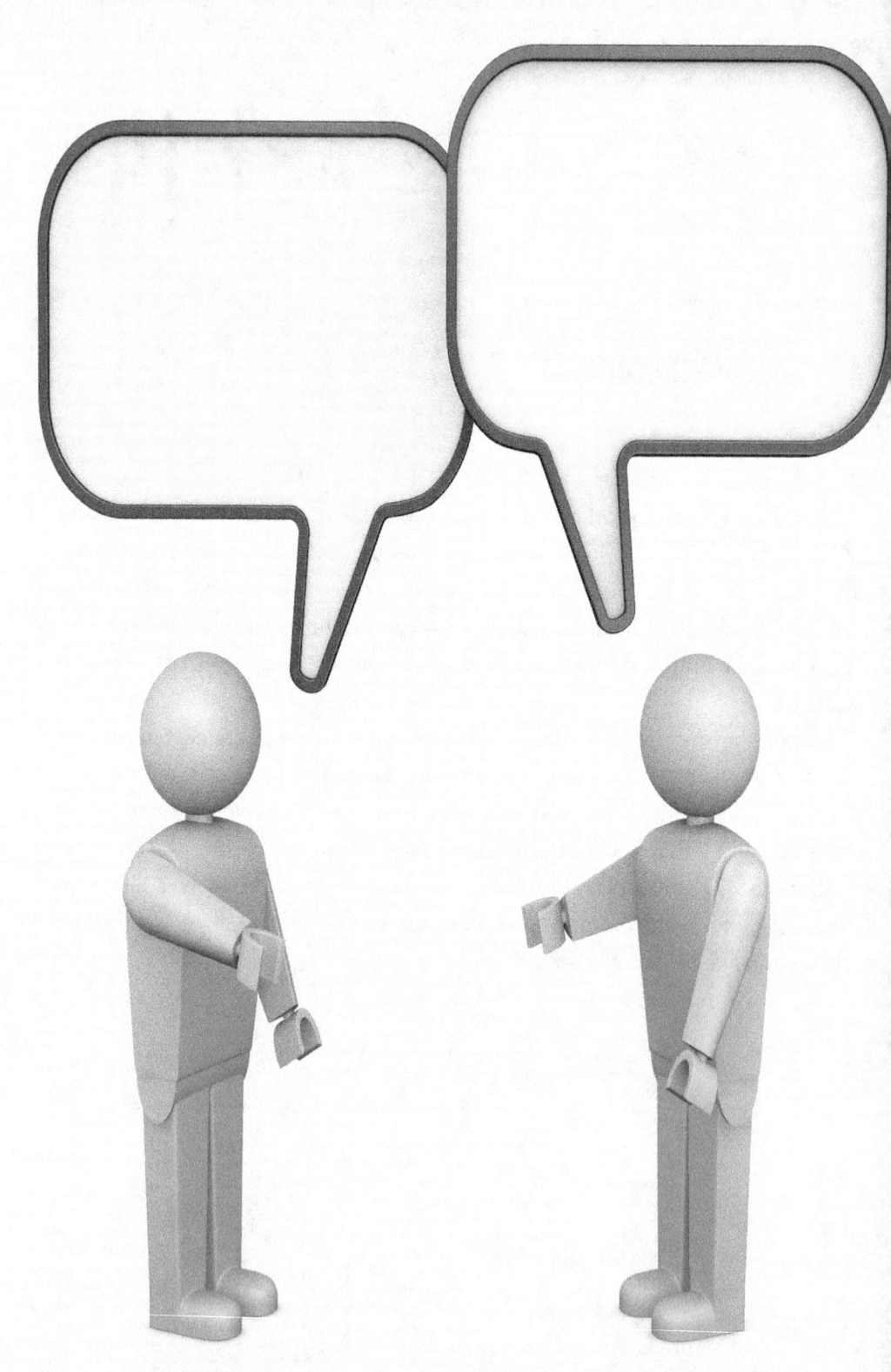

16

Talk is not cheap.

Don't be afraid to share your success with other people. This does not mean discussing it every waking hour. It does mean that dialogue with friends and co-workers will reinforce your commitment to your lifestyle while giving them the opportunity to jump on board. It is important to be selective with when and how you bring it up. It should not be an opportunity to brag; it should be an opportunity to inform. It should not be an opportunity to create boredom; it should be an opportunity to stimulate.

To recap what we have covered: experience your **pivotal moment** and then set in motion **sustainable weight loss for a lifetime**. The sixteen helpful guidelines are as follows:

1. Be in control of what you eat and how you order your food.

2. If you snack, cut food into small portions.

3. Drink water.

4. Eat a healthy breakfast. Include a protein shake.

5. Don't deny yourself specific food groups.

6. Eat foods plain without all the calorie-loaded toppings.

7. Avoid grease.

8. Eat the type of foods you enjoy in smaller bites.

9. Exercise – walk or run for success. Add weight training and core strengthening for muscle toning.

10. Take your time losing weight. Appreciate small changes.

11. Use smart flavorings in and on your food.

12. Avoid empty calories, and added sugar or salt.

13. Make good choices and select appropriate portion size.

14. Lifetime companions—limit stress, get a good night's sleep, take a multivitamin, ensure good dental hygiene, and take time off for you.

15. Cross over to your new lifestyle.

16. Don't be afraid to share your success.

Important Appendices to Follow

Appendix A

Fitness Workout

Weight Training Regimen

Begin with a series of stretching exercises. Then perform a fifteen minute cardio workout on the treadmill. Now you are ready to move into weight training, with 2-3 sets of the following exercises.

1. Seated Leg Press – 15 reps
2. Floor Ball – Hamstring Curl-ins 30 reps
3. Lateral Pull Downs – 15 reps
4. Compound Rows – 15 reps
5. Vertical Chest – 15 reps
6. Floor Exercise – Pushups, 30 seconds
7. Abdominal Floor Roller – 15 reps
8. Floor Exercise – Planks, 30 seconds
9. Overhead Press – 15 reps
10. Renegade Rows – Floor Exercise – 30 reps, 15 lb. square hand Weights

(Adapt the amount of weight in the above exercises to your capabilities)

Cardio Regimens

Treadmill – 5 minute warm-up at a lower speed.

55 minutes at higher speeds and incline.

Or

20/20/20/ Rotation

Rotate through 20 minutes on each of three machines (treadmill, recumbent bike, and elliptical)

Begin the Cardio Regimen with a series of stretching exercises and finish with a fifteen minute series of weight training exercises to work your upper body and abdominals.

Core Strengthening Regimen

Begin with a series of stretching exercises. Then move to the core strengthening exercises in a quantity and duration that matches your ability.

1. Pushups
2. Front Plank
3. Side Planks
4. Leg Lifts - Elevate 6 inches above the floor and hold.
5. Half Sit-ups - lift part way off the floor and hold.
6. Floor Ball – Place feet and lower legs over the floor ball. Elevate your back off the floor and curl the ball into your buttocks.
7. Renegade Rows – While prone to the floor and elevated above square hand weights, alternate drawing each weight into your chest and then back down to the floor.
8. Abdominal Floor Roller
9. Lateral Pull Downs – Weight training machine
10. Seated Leg Press – Weight training machine

The prior workouts are intended as an example. Any workout routine should be reviewed by your trainer and adapted to you as an individual. These workouts are just a few of the many possibilities for a fitness training regimen. Set a routine for your workout sessions but in all likelihood you will not be able to make every session every week. Two or three good workouts each week with stretching/core strengthening in between, at the gym or home, is a good mix. Then enjoy the weekend and give your body a rest. There will be personal and work-related events that will require your time. Keep the routine, even though there will be holes in it from time to time.

In addition, it is very important to communicate with your trainer after the first couple of sessions to fine tune your workout routine that you can easily duplicate on the days the trainer is not working with you. Eventually you will be ready to "fly" on your own. To create an effective routine there must be a great deal of communication between you and your trainer—each individual has a different body and no single routine will be right for everyone. Remember: **"slow and in control, "pace the weights,"** and **"listen to your body."**

Appendix B

Weight Record (approximately eighteen months)

4/7 222 lbs.
  (Physician office records)

7/12 212 lbs.
  (Three month check)

8/13 210 lbs.
  (Begin weekly weighing)
8/20 208.5 lbs.
8/27 207.0 lbs.

9/3 205.0 lbs.
9/9 203.0 lbs.
9/26 202.5 lbs.

10/1 200.5 lbs.
10/8 199.0 lbs.
  (Break through plateau)
10/15 199.0 lbs.
10/22 196.0 lbs.
10/29 196.5 lbs.

11/4 193.0 lbs.
11/12 194.0 lbs.
  (Bump up -this
  will happen)
11/19 193.5 lbs.
11/26 193.5 lbs.

12/3 190.5 lbs
12/10 190.5 lbs.
12/17 189.0 lbs.
  (Break through plateau)
12/24 187.5 lbs.
12/31 188.5 lbs.

1/14 187.5 lbs.
1/22 192.5 lbs.
  (Vacation – Too much food/
  drinks and
  salty foods)
1/28 187.0 lbs.

2/4 187.0 lbs.
2/10 186.0 lbs.

2/18 187.5 lbs.
2/25 188.0 lbs.
   (Bump up- this will happen)

3/5 185.5 lbs.
3/12 186.5 lbs.
3/18 184.5 lbs.
3/25 184.5 lbs.

4/1 183.5 lbs.
4/8 181.5 lbs.
4/15 181.0 lbs.
4/22 181.0 lbs.
4/29 183.0 lbs.
   (Bump up-this will happen)

5/5 180.0 lbs.
5/12 180.0 lbs.
5/20 181.0 lbs.
5/27 179.5 lbs.
   (Break through plateau)

6/3 179.0 lbs.
6/10 178.5 lbs.
6/17 178.0 lbs.
6/24 177.0 lbs.
6/30 179.0 lbs.

7/8 176.0 lbs.
7/15 177.0 lbs.
7/22 176.0 lbs.
7/29 176.0 lbs.

8/6 175.0 lbs.
8/11 175.5 lbs.
8/19 176.5 lbs.
8/26 178.0 lbs.

9/2 176.0 lbs.
9/9 176.0 lbs.
9/16 175 lbs.
   (Target weight achieved and
   held for over six months as
   of this printing.)

Appendix C

Weight Chart

Since this book is a working tool, the following pages are included for your use in charting your weight to a successful conclusion.

Week	Date	Weight
Week 1		
Week 2		
Week 3		
Week 4		
Week 5		
Week 6		
Week 7		
Week 8		
Week 9		
Week 10		
Week 11		
Week 12		
Week 13		
Week 14		

Notes

Week	Date	Weight
Week 15		
Week 16		
Week 17		
Week 18		
Week 19		
Week 20		
Week 21		
Week 22		
Week 23		
Week 24		
Week 25		
Week 26		
Week 27		
Week 28		
Week 29		
Week 30		
Week 31		
Week 32		
Week 33		
Week 34		
Week 35		

Notes

Week	Date	Weight
Week 36		
Week 37		
Week 38		
Week 39		
Week 40		
Week 41		
Week 42		
Week 43		
Week 44		
Week 45		
Week 46		
Week 47		
Week 48		
Week 49		
Week 50		
Week 51		
Week 52		

Congratulations!

Notes

Appendix D

Fitness chart

You will diversify and make changes to your workout routines over time. The following pages are included to chart those changes.

Routine 1

Routine 2

Routine 3

Routine 4

Routine 5